MEDITERRANEAN DIET COOKBOOK

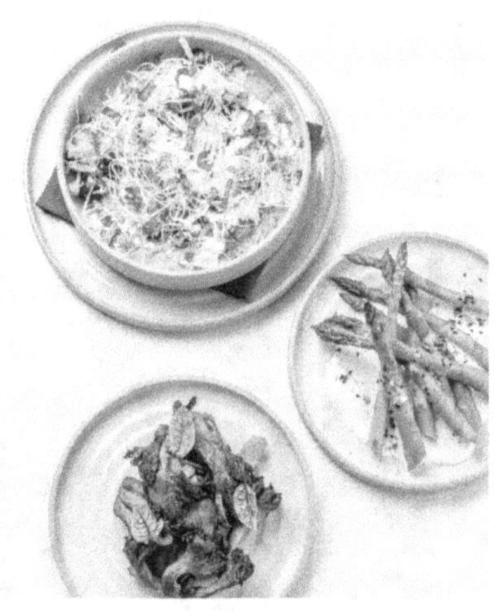

Delicious And Flavorful Recipes For Health And Wellness While Embracing The Mediterranean Lifestyle

Hannah Pullman

GAIN ACCESS TO MORE BOOKS FROM ME

Table of Contents

Introduction
　　Overview of the Mediterranean Diet
　　Health Benefits
Essential Ingredients
　　Olive Oil
　　A primary source of beneficial monounsaturated fats.
　　Vegetables and Fruits
　　Whole Grains
　　Fish and Seafood
　　Seeds and Nuts
　　Spices and Herbs
　　Wine (not required)
　　Water
　　Lean proteins
　　Legumes
Breakfast Delights
　　Greek Yogurt Parfait
　　Mediterranean Omelet
　　Whole Grain Pancakes with Berries
Appetizers and Mezes
　　Hummus and Pita Bread
　　Stuffed Grape Leaves
　　Roasted Red Pepper and Feta Dip
Fresh Salads

Greek Salad

Caprese salad

Quinoa and Chickpea Salad

Main Courses

Mediterranean Baked Fish

Lemon Herb Chicken Skewers

Eggplant Parmesan

Vegetarian Delights

Ratatouille

Lentil and Vegetable Stew

Spinach and Feta Stuffed Peppers

Sides and Accompaniments

Sauce Tzatziki

Roasted Vegetables with Herbs

Couscous with Pine Nuts

Desserts

Fresh Fruit Sorbet

Olive Oil and Orange Cake

Honey and Nut Baklava

Lifestyle Tips

Tips for Grocery Shopping

Physical Activity and the Mediterranean Lifestyle

7-Days Meal Plan

Sample Weekly Menu

Conclusion

Encouragement for a Healthier Lifestyle

Introduction

Greetings from the Mediterranean diet cookbook universe! The Mediterranean region's unique flavors and health advantages are highlighted in this cooking guide. Discover an abundance of dishes that highlight lean proteins, nutritious grains, fresh veggies, and olive oil. Prepare yourself for a delectable voyage through the colorful and varied cuisine of the Mediterranean that supports heart health and general well-being.

Overview of the Mediterranean Diet

The traditional eating habits of the Mediterranean Diet are derived from the nations that border the Mediterranean Sea. It highlights:

1. Plant-Based Foods: The cornerstone consists of fruits, vegetables, whole grains, legumes, and nuts.

2.Healthy Fats: Monounsaturated fats, which are found in olive oil, are the main type of fat.

3. Lean Proteins: Instead of red meat, choose beans, fish, and fowl. Fish is a staple food that is particularly high in omega-3 fatty acids.

4. Dairy: Moderate intake of yogurt and cheese, frequently in fermented varieties.

5. Herbs and Spices: Mediterranean cuisines employ herbs and spices to provide flavor instead of salt.

6. Moderate Wine Consumption: Red wine is linked to a diet when it is used in moderation.

7. Physical Activity: It's well accepted that regular exercise is essential to a healthy lifestyle.

The potential health benefits of the Mediterranean diet are well known, and these include improved heart health, weight management, and general wellbeing.

Health Benefits

Numerous health advantages are linked to the Mediterranean diet, such as:

1. Heart Health: Olive oil, which is high in heart-healthy monounsaturated fats, may lower the risk of heart disease.

2. Weight Management: Putting a focus on whole grains, fruits, and vegetables can help with weight management.

3. Cancer Prevention: Eating foods high in antioxidants, such as fruits and vegetables, may help reduce the chance of developing some types of cancer.

4.Brain Health: Fish oil, which contains omega-3 fatty acids, may improve cognitive performance and lower the risk of cognitive decline.

5.Management of Diabetes: The diet's emphasis on lean proteins, beans, and whole grains may help control blood sugar levels.

6. Inflammation Reduction: Fish and olive oil, which are anti-inflammatory foods, may aid in the fight against chronic inflammation.

7.Longevity: Research indicates that following the Mediterranean diet may extend one's life.

Recall that every person will react differently, and that leading a balanced lifestyle is crucial for general wellbeing.

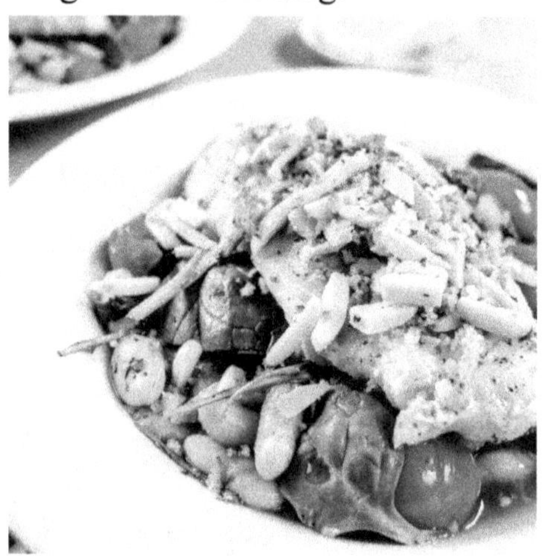

Essential Ingredients

The Mediterranean Diet emphasizes:

Olive Oil

A primary source of beneficial monounsaturated fats.

Vegetables and Fruits

Add a range of vibrant vegetables, citrus fruits, olives, tomatoes, and leafy greens.

Whole Grains

For instance, whole wheat bread and brown rice

Fish and Seafood

rich in heart-healthy omega-3 fatty acids.

Seeds and Nuts

Give them fiber, protein, and healthy fats.

Spices and Herbs

savory salt substitutes that lower sodium consumption.

Wine (not required)

Red wine may be beneficial to the heart when consumed in moderation.

Water

Hydration is vital to general well-being.

Lean proteins

Eggs, dairy products, and poultry in moderation

Legumes

For protein and fiber, try beans, lentils, and chickpeas.

Recall that the Mediterranean Diet encourages eating in a diversified and balanced manner.

Breakfast Delights

Indulge in a Mediterranean-inspired breakfast:

Greek Yogurt Parfait

This is a basic recipe for a parfait made using Greek yogurt:

Ingredients:
1 cup of unsweetened Greek yogurt
A half-cup of fresh berries, such as raspberries, strawberries, or blueberries
1/4 cup of finely chopped nuts (walnuts or almonds)
One tablespoon of honey
1/4 cup granola, if desired
One teaspoon of optional chia seeds

Instructions:
1. Spread Greek yogurt at the bottom of a serving glass or bowl.

2.Scatter some fresh berries over the yogurt.

3. Toss in chopped nuts for extra crunch and heart-healthy fats when you sprinkle the berries.

4. For a touch of sweetness, drizzle honey over the layers.

5. You can add granola for extra texture if you'd like.

6. You can optionally add chia seeds for added nutritious value.

7. Continue layering until you reach the top, then sprinkle more honey on top.

Enjoy a tasty Greek yogurt parfait that complies with the Mediterranean Diet's focus on whole, fresh foods by serving it right away.

Mediterranean Omelet

The following is a quick and easy recipe for Mediterranean omelets:

Ingredients:

three big eggs

one-fourth cup of chopped tomatoes

1/4 cup of finely chopped spinach

1/4 cup chopped bell peppers, ideally yellow or red

Two teaspoons of crumbled feta cheese

One tablespoon of olive oil

One-half tsp dried oregano

To taste, add salt and pepper.

Instructions:

1. Whisk eggs, oregano, salt, and pepper in a bowl.

2. Heat the olive oil in a nonstick skillet over medium heat.

3. Fill the skillet with diced bell peppers, diced tomatoes, and chopped spinach. Sauté the veggies till they get soft.

4. Cover the skillet's sautéed vegetables with the whisked eggs.

5.Leave the eggs to set slightly on the rims, and then use a spatula to gently whisk the mixture.

6. Evenly scatter the crumbled feta cheese over the omelet once the eggs are mostly done but still a little runny on top.

7. After folding the omelet in half, cook it for one more minute, or until the eggs are done.

8. Transfer the warm Mediterranean omelet to a platter.

Savor your flavorful and nutrient-dense Mediterranean omelet!

Whole Grain Pancakes with Berries

This is a straightforward recipe that fits the Mediterranean Diet for whole grain pancakes with berries:

Ingredients:
1 cup flour (whole wheat).
One spoonful of maple syrup or honey
One tsp baking powder
One-half tsp baking soda
1/4 tsp salt

One cup of Greek yogurt

2/3 cup milk (for a dairy-free option, use almond milk)

One big egg

One tsp vanilla essence

Blueberries, strawberries, and raspberries combined for the garnish

Instructions:

1. Combine the whole wheat flour, baking soda, baking powder, and salt in a sizable bowl.

2. Gently stir together the Greek yogurt, milk, egg, vanilla extract, and honey (or maple syrup) in a separate bowl.

3. Add the wet mixture to the dry mixture and whisk just until blended. Take care not to overmix; a little lumpiness in the batter is acceptable.

4. Turn up the heat to medium on a nonstick skillet or griddle. Apply a little layer of cooking spray or a tiny bit of oil.

5. For each pancake, pour 1/4 cup of batter onto the griddle. Cook until surface bubbles appear,

then turn and continue cooking until golden brown on the other side.

6.Continue till the batter is used up.

7. Present the pancakes with an abundance of mixed berries on top.

Savor your tasty and wholesome whole grain pancakes with berries, which are a great fit for the Mediterranean diet!

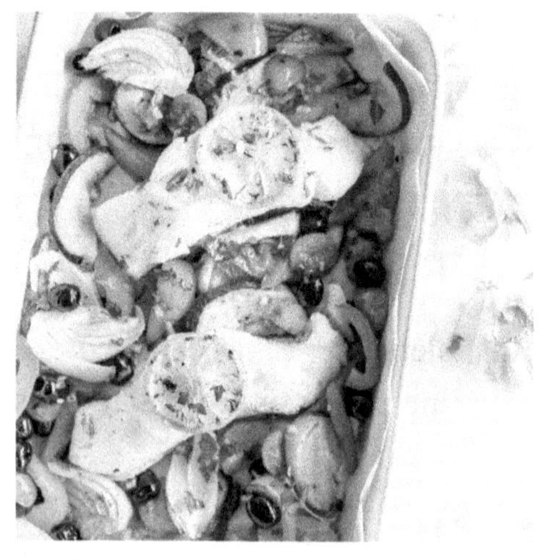

Appetizers and Mezes

Certainly! Mediterranean cuisine offers a variety of delicious appetizers and mezes. Consider options like:

Hummus and Pita Bread

This is a quick and easy Mediterranean-style hummus and pita bread recipe:

Hummus:
Ingredients:
One can (15 oz) of rinsed and drained chickpeas
One-fourth cup tahini
One-fourth cup of extra virgin olive oil
one minced clove of garlic
two tsp lemon juice
half a teaspoon of cumin powder
To taste, add salt and pepper. Water (as needed for consistency)

Instructions:
1. Place the chickpeas, tahini, olive oil, garlic, lemon juice, cumin, salt, and pepper in a food processor.

2. Blend until smooth, adding water as necessary to get the consistency you want.

3. Taste and adjust seasonings.

Pita Bread:
2 1/4 teaspoons sugar, 1 teaspoon active dry yeast, 1 cup warm water, and 3 cups all-purpose flour
One tablespoon olive oil and one teaspoon salt

Instructional:
1. Combine yeast, sugar, and warm water in a bowl. Until foamy, let it sit for five to ten minutes.

2. Mix the flour and salt together in a sizable mixing basin. Create a well in the middle and pour in the olive oil and yeast mixture.

3. Mix until a dough forms, then knead for about five minutes, or until smooth, on a floured surface.

4.Stand the dough in a bowl that has been lightly oiled, cover it with a damp cloth, and let it rise in a warm location until it has doubled in size, about an hour.

5.Set the oven's temperature to 475°F (245°C).

6. Flatten the dough and form it into tiny spheres. Shape every ball into a slender circle.

7.Send the circles to bake on a baking sheet for 5 to 7 minutes, or until they are gently golden and puffy.

Savor your pita bread and homemade hummus!

Stuffed Grape Leaves

This is a straightforward recipe for filled grape leaves, a traditional Mediterranean meal:

Ingredients:

1/2 cup olive oil and 1 cup uncooked short-grain rice
One large onion, diced finely
two minced garlic cloves
half a cup of pine nuts
half a cup of raisins or currants
One teaspoon of cinnamon powder
One teaspoon of allspice powder
To taste, add salt and pepper.
half a cup of freshly chopped parsley
one-fourth cup of finely chopped fresh mint
One jar of brined grape leaves, rinsed and drained
Two lemons, to be juiced

Instructions:

1. Prepare the rice per the directions on the package.

2. In a skillet, soften and transparently sauté the minced garlic and diced onion in olive oil.

3. Toss in the pine nuts and toast them in the pan until they start to turn golden brown.

4. Add the cooked rice, salt, pepper, ground cinnamon, ground allspice, and currants or raisins. Blend thoroughly.

5. Turn off the heat source and allow the mixture to cool. After the mixture cools down, thoroughly stir in the chopped parsley and mint.

6. With the shiny side facing down, take a grape leaf and press a tiny bit of the rice mixture into the middle. Roll it tightly after folding the sides over the filling.

7. Tightly put the packed grape leaves into a big pot, seam side down.

8. Drizzle the filled grape leaves with the juice of two lemons.

9. Fill the pot with water until the grape leaves are barely submerged.

10. To prevent the grape leaves from unfolding while they cook, place a heavy dish on top of them.

11. After bringing the water to a boil, lower the heat to a simmer, cover, and cook the rice for 45 to 1 hour, depending on how done it is.

12. Before serving, let the filled grape leaves cool.

Savor your mouthwatering stuffed grape leaves—a savory and nourishing addition to any Mediterranean diet.

Roasted Red Pepper and Feta Dip

This is a straightforward Mediterranean-style recipe for Roasted Red Pepper and Feta Dip:

Ingredients:
Two big red bell peppers
One cup of feta cheese, crumbled
One-fourth cup of extra virgin olive oil
two minced garlic cloves
One tablespoon of lemon juice
One tsp of dehydrated oregano
To taste, add salt and pepper.
Not required: As a garnish, use fresh parsley.

Instructions:

1. Set oven temperature to 400°F, or 200°C. After placing the full red bell peppers on a baking sheet, roast them for about 25 to 30 minutes, rotating them occasionally, until the skins are blistered and browned.

2. Take out of the oven and transfer the peppers to a bowl. Place a plastic wrap over the bowl and allow it to cool. After the peppers have cooled, cut them into pieces and take off the skins and seeds.

3.Place the feta crumbles, olive oil, chopped garlic, lemon juice, and dry oregano in a food processor. Process till smooth.

4. To taste, add salt and pepper to the dip. If necessary, adjust the consistency by adding extra olive oil.

5. Spoon the dip into a dish for serving. Add fresh parsley as a garnish if you'd like.

6. You can serve the Roasted Red Pepper and Feta Dip with cucumber slices, whole-grain pita bread, or any other vegetables of your choice.

Savor your tasty dip with a hint of Mediterranean flavor!

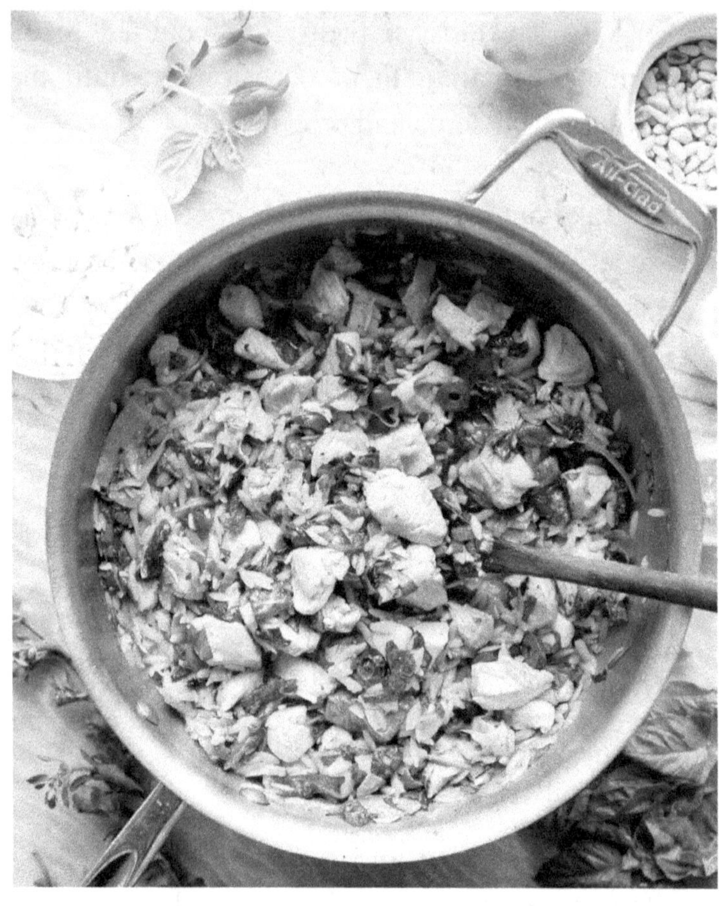

Fresh Salads

Here are some simple Mediterranean-inspired salad recipes:

Greek Salad

Here's a basic Greek salad dish with Mediterranean influences:

Ingredients:
diced 1 cup Kalamata olives, diced 1 cucumber, diced 1 red onion, diced 1 green bell pepper, pitted 200g feta cheese, crumbled
One-fourth cup of extra virgin olive oil
Two tsp red wine vinegar
One tsp of dehydrated oregano
To taste, add salt and pepper.

Instructions:
1. Combine the tomatoes, bell pepper, cucumber, red onion, and olives in a large bowl.

2. To make the dressing, combine the olive oil, red wine vinegar, oregano, salt, and pepper in a another bowl.

3.Add the salad dressing and gently mix to coat the veggies.

4. Top the salad with a sprinkle of feta cheese.

5. To enable the flavors to mingle, refrigerate for at least half an hour before serving.

Savor your crisp Greek salad, a tasty and nourishing choice for a Mediterranean lifestyle.

Caprese salad

This is a straightforward recipe for caprese salad that fits into the Mediterranean diet:

Ingredients:
4 large, sliced ripe tomatoes
One pound of freshly sliced mozzarella cheese
fresh leaves of basil
Extra virgin olive oil
vinegar with balsamic
To taste, add salt and pepper.

Instructions:

1. Arrange the tomato and mozzarella slices in an alternating fashion on a serving plate.

2. Sandwich the tomato and mozzarella slices between a few fresh basil leaves.

3. Balsamic vinegar and extra virgin olive oil should be drizzled over the salad.

4. Add pepper and salt to taste.

In order to savor the freshness, serve right away. This recipe encourages a healthy and balanced eating style because it is full of complete, fresh ingredients that are often seen in the Mediterranean diet.

Quinoa and Chickpea Salad

This is a straightforward recipe for chickpea and quinoa salad that fits the Mediterranean diet:

Ingredients:
2 cups water and 1 cup washed quinoa
one cup (15 oz) of chickpeas, one cucumber, one cup diced cherry tomatoes, one half red

onion, one cup chopped coarsely, one cup feta cheese, sliced, and one cup Kalamata olives
1/4 cup finely chopped fresh parsley

For the Dressing:
One-fourth cup of extra virgin olive oil
Two tsp red wine vinegar
One tsp of dehydrated oregano
To taste, add salt and pepper.

Instructions:
1. Combine water and quinoa in a medium pot. After bringing to a boil, lower the heat, cover, and simmer the quinoa for 15 to 20 minutes, or until it is tender and the water has been absorbed. Using a fork, fluff and allow to cool.

2.Combine the cooked quinoa, cucumber, cherry tomatoes, red onion, olives, feta cheese, parsley, and chickpeas in a big bowl.

3. Combine the olive oil, red wine vinegar, salt, pepper, and dried oregano in a small bowl. After adding the dressing to the salad, gently toss to mix.

4. To let the flavors to mingle, refrigerate for a minimum of half an hour.

Enjoy your flavorful Mediterranean quinoa and chickpea salad, served cold!
This recipe emphasizes whole grains, legumes, veggies, and healthy fats, all of which are in line with the tenets of the Mediterranean diet.

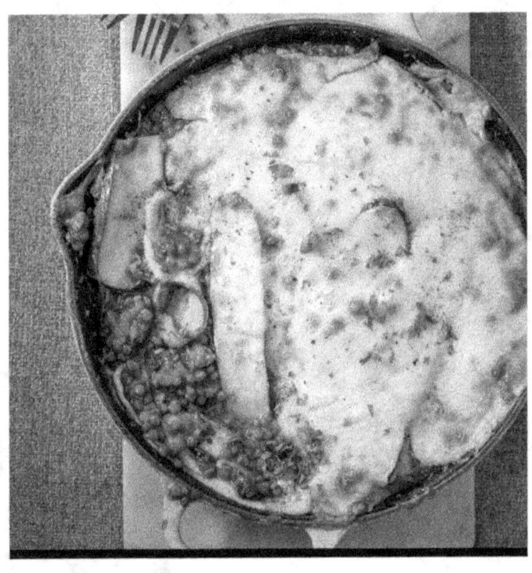

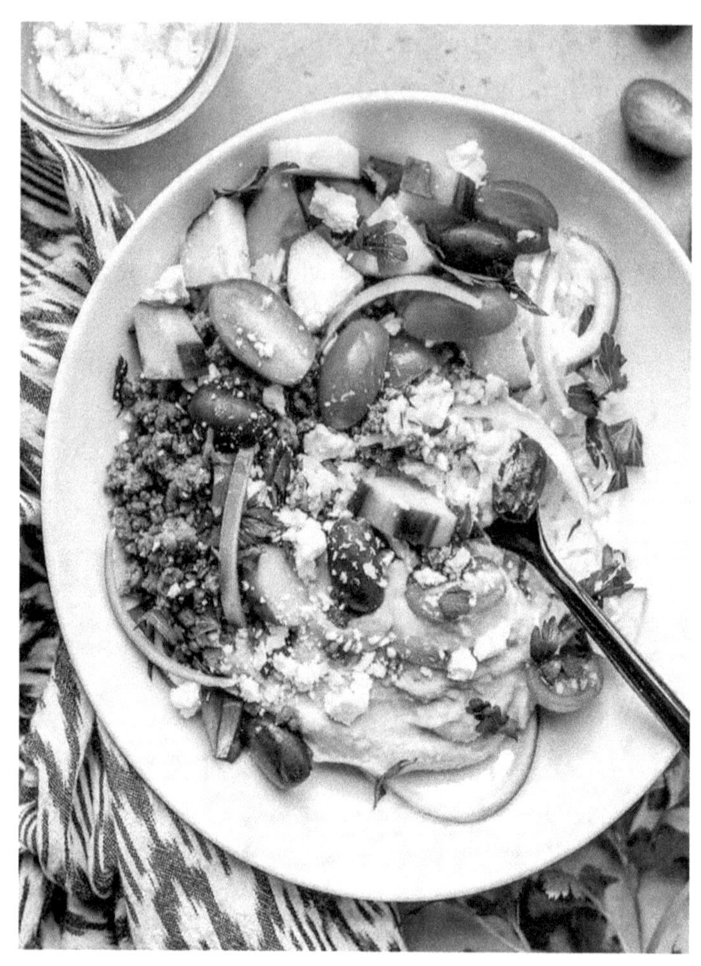

Main Courses

Here are a few main course recipes that follow the Mediterranean diet's guidelines:

Mediterranean Baked Fish

This is a quick and tasty baked fish recipe that fits within the Mediterranean diet:

Ingredients:
Four fish filets (such as tilapia or cod) are the ingredients.
1 sliced lemon
Two tsp olive oil
three minced garlic cloves
One tsp of dehydrated oregano
A single tsp of dried thyme
One tsp of dehydrated rosemary
To taste, add salt and pepper.
Half a cup of cherry tomatoes
One-fourth cup sliced Kalamata olives and two teaspoons capers

Instructions:
Set the oven temperature to 375°F, or 190°C.

2. Transfer the fish fillets to an ovenproof dish.

3. Coat the filets with olive oil and massage them with finely chopped garlic.

4. Top the fish with a sprinkle of salt, pepper, thyme, and oregano.

5. Place a few slices of lemon over the filets.

6. Arrange capers, Kalamata olives, and cherry tomatoes all around the fish.

7. Bake the fish for 20 to 25 minutes, or until it is cooked through and flakes readily with a fork, in a preheated oven.

8. Present the cooked fish beside the pan juices and roasted veggies.

This dish, which emphasizes fresh ingredients, herbs, and olive oil, is not only delicious but also follows the guidelines of the Mediterranean diet. Savor your food!

Lemon Herb Chicken Skewers

This is a straightforward Lemon Herb Chicken Skewer dish that is suitable for a Mediterranean diet:

Ingredients:
1.5 pounds of chopped, skinless, boneless chicken breasts
two lemons, both juiced and zesty
three minced garlic cloves
Two tablespoons of freshly chopped oregano
Two tablespoons of freshly chopped parsley
A single tsp of dried thyme
Two tsp olive oil
To taste, add salt and pepper.
Water-soaked wooden skewers

Instructions:
1. Combine the lemon zest, lemon juice, olive oil, salt, pepper, minced garlic, chopped oregano, parsley, and dried thyme in a bowl. This marinade is what you'll use.

2. Make sure the chicken chunks are thoroughly coated by placing them in the marinade. For

maximum taste, marinate for at least 30 minutes or overnight covered and chilled.

3. Set the temperature on your oven or grill to medium-high.

4. Thread the moistened wooden skewers with the marinated chicken.

5. Cook the skewers, rotating them from time to time, for ten to fifteen minutes, or until the chicken is thoroughly cooked and nicely charred.

6. For a whole Mediterranean-style dinner, serve the Lemon Herb Chicken Skewers with cherry tomatoes, mixed greens, and a drizzle of olive oil.

Savor your tasty and healthful chicken skewers with a Mediterranean flair!

Eggplant Parmesan

This is a straightforward Mediterranean-style eggplant parmesan recipe:

Ingredients:
1/2-inch circles cut from one big eggplant
two beaten eggs
One cup breadcrumbs made from whole wheat
Grated Parmesan cheese, one cup
Two cups of homemade tomato sauce with olive oil
One cup of shredded mozzarella cheese
two teaspoons finely chopped fresh basil
Two tsp olive oil
To taste, add salt and pepper.

Instructions:
1.Set the oven temperature to 375°F, or 190°C.

2. To remove extra moisture, sprinkle salt on the eggplant slices and let them sit for 30 minutes. After that, blot them dry using a paper towel.

3. Combine breadcrumbs and Parmesan cheese in a small bowl. Coat each eggplant slice with the breadcrumb mixture after dipping it into the beaten eggs.

4. In a skillet over medium heat, preheat the olive oil.

5. Cook each side of the breaded eggplant slices until golden brown. To absorb excess oil, place them on a paper towel.

6. Evenly cover the baking dish with tomato sauce. Scatter the cooked eggplant slices on top in a layer.

7. Garnish with chopped basil and mozzarella cheese. Continue layering ingredients until all are utilized, and then top with a layer of cheese and basil.

8. Bake for 25 to 30 minutes, or until the cheese is bubbling and melted, in a preheated oven.

Let it cool for a few minutes before serving. Savor your eggplant parmesan in a Mediterranean manner.

Vegetarian Delights

The following vegetarian meals follow the guidelines of the Mediterranean diet:

Ratatouille

This is a straightforward recipe for Ratatouille that fits into the Mediterranean diet:

Ingredients:
2 cloves of finely chopped garlic, minced 4 tomatoes, diced 1 eggplant, diced 1 zucchini, diced 1 yellow bell pepper, diced 1 red bell pepper, diced 1 onion
two Tablespoons tomato paste
One tsp of dehydrated oregano
A single tsp of dried thyme
One-fourth cup of extra virgin olive oil
To taste, add salt and pepper.
For garnish, use fresh basil.

Instructions:
1. Turn the oven on to 375°F, or 190°C.

2. Combine the diced eggplant, zucchini, bell peppers, onion, and garlic in a sizable baking dish.

3.Combine the diced tomatoes, tomato paste, olive oil, thyme, oregano, and pepper in another bowl.

4.Coat the vegetables equally by pouring the tomato mixture over them in the baking dish and tossing everything together.

5. Bake, stirring halfway through, in the preheated oven for 45 to 50 minutes, or until the veggies are soft.

6. After cooking, take it out of the oven and allow it to cool somewhat. Add some fresh basil as a garnish before serving.

In addition to being tasty, this Ratatouille is loaded with the vibrant, nutrient-dense veggies that are a staple of the Mediterranean diet. Have fun!

Lentil and Vegetable Stew

This is a tasty stew of lentils and vegetables that is appropriate for a Mediterranean diet:

Ingredients:
1 cup washed brown or green lentils
Two tsp olive oil
One chopped onion, two chopped carrots, two chopped celery stalks, and three minced garlic cloves
One can, or fourteen ounces chopped tomatoes
One tsp of dehydrated oregano
One teaspoon each of ground cumin and dried thyme
Four cups of broth made with vegetables
One chopped zucchini
One sliced red bell pepper and one cup of chopped kale or greens
To taste, add salt and pepper.
As a garnish, use fresh parsley.

Instructions:
1. Heat the olive oil in a big pot over medium heat. Saute the onions, carrots, and celery until they are soft.

2. Add the minced garlic and stir until fragrant, about 1 more minute.

3. Add the cumin, thyme, oregano, and diced tomatoes. Allow the flavors to mingle by cooking for five minutes.

4. Add the veggie broth and the rinsed lentils. After bringing to a boil, lower the heat, cover, and simmer the lentils for 20 to 25 minutes, or until they are soft.

5. Add chopped kale or spinach, red bell pepper, and zucchini. After ten more minutes of simmering, the vegetables should be soft.

6. Season to taste with salt and pepper. If necessary, adjust the herbs.

7. Garnish the hot lentil and vegetable stew with fresh parsley.

This filling and healthy stew, which has a lot of veggies, lentils, and olive oil, follows the guidelines of the Mediterranean diet.

Spinach and Feta Stuffed Peppers

This is a straightforward recipe for spinach and feta-stuffed peppers that complies with the guidelines of the Mediterranean diet:

Ingredients:
Four sizable bell peppers, any color will do
One cup of cooked quinoa
1/2 cup of crumbled feta cheese and one cup of freshly chopped spinach
1/4 cup chopped sun-dried tomatoes, 1/4 cup chopped Kalamata olives, minced garlic cloves, and 1 teaspoon dried oregano
To taste, add salt and pepper.
Use olive oil to drizzle

Instructions:
1. Turn the oven on to 375°F, or 190°C.

2. Cut the bell peppers' tops off, removing the seeds and membranes.

3.Combine the cooked quinoa, chopped spinach, feta cheese, sun-dried tomatoes, olives, minced garlic, oregano, salt, and pepper in a sizable mixing dish.

4. Carefully put the quinoa mixture into each bell pepper.

5. Transfer the filled peppers to a baking tray and drizzle with olive oil.

6. Bake the peppers for 25 to 30 minutes, or until they are soft, in a preheated oven.

7. Present the filled peppers hot, topped with extra feta cheese and, if preferred, a dash of oregano.

Savor your tasty and nourishing dinner with a Mediterranean flair!

Sides and Accompaniments

Consider the following sides and accompaniments for a Mediterranean diet:

Sauce Tzatziki

This is a straightforward Mediterranean-style Tzatziki Sauce recipe:

Ingredients:
1 thinly sliced cucumber
two cups of Greek yogurt
two minced garlic cloves
One tablespoon of olive oil
One tablespoon of freshly chopped dill
One tablespoon of freshly chopped mint
To taste, add salt and pepper.
Lemon juice (extra virgin olive oil optional)

Instructions:
1. Using a fresh kitchen towel, grate the cucumber and squeeze out any extra water.

2. Combine the grated cucumber, Greek yogurt, olive oil, chopped garlic, mint, dill, and salt and pepper in a bowl.

3. Thoroughly mix until all components are combined.

4. Taste and adjust the seasoning, adding a dash of lemon juice if preferred.

5.To let the flavors to mingle, let it cool in the fridge for at least half an hour.

Savor the crisp and healthful addition of your own Tzatziki Sauce to your Mediterranean-inspired dishes!

Roasted Vegetables with Herbs

This is a quick and tasty dish for roasted veggies with herbs that goes well with a Mediterranean diet:

Ingredients:
1 sliced zucchini
One red bell pepper, thinly sliced

One yellow bell pepper, thinly sliced
One sliced red onion
One cup of cherry tomatoes
Two tsp olive oil
One tsp of dehydrated oregano
A single tsp of dried thyme
One tsp of dehydrated rosemary
To taste, add salt and pepper.

Instructions:
Set the oven's temperature to 425°F (220°C).

2. Combine the bell peppers, cherry tomatoes, zucchini slices, and red onion in a big bowl and mix with olive oil.

3. Top the vegetables with a sprinkle of salt, pepper, dried oregano, thyme, and rosemary. Mix well until the flavors and herbs are uniformly distributed throughout the veggies.

4. Arrange the seasoned veggies in a single layer on a parchment paper-lined baking sheet.

5. Roast, stirring halfway through, in a preheated oven for 25 to 30 minutes, or until the veggies are soft and beginning to caramelize.

6. Take it out of the oven and let it to cool down a little before serving.

Savor the flavor of your herb-roasted Mediterranean veggies!

Couscous with Pine Nuts

This dish for couscous with pine nuts is tasty and healthy, making it a great fit for the Mediterranean diet:

Ingredients:
2 teaspoons olive oil, 1 1/4 cups vegetable broth, and 1 cup couscous.
half a cup of almonds
One little red onion, cut finely
One cup cherry tomatoes, cut in half, two minced garlic cloves, and half a cup diced cucumber
1/4 cup of freshly chopped parsley and 1/4 cup of freshly chopped mint
To taste, add salt and pepper.
slices of lemon for serving

Instructions:

1.In a saucepan, bring the vegetable broth to a boil. Remove from heat, cover, and stir in the couscous. Use a fork to fluff it after five minutes.

2.Over medium heat, preheat the olive oil in a skillet. Add the pine nuts and toast, stirring often, until golden brown. Take out and place aside from the skillet.

3.Add minced garlic and chopped red onion to the same skillet. Sauté the food until it becomes tender.

4.In a big bowl, mix the cooked couscous, toasted pine nuts, cherry tomatoes, cucumber, parsley, and mint along with the sautéed onion and garlic.

5.Season with salt and pepper to taste and drizzle with more olive oil. Mix everything until thoroughly incorporated.

6.You can serve the chilled or room temperature couscous combination. Add some lemon wedges as a garnish for a taste explosion.

This dish for couscous with pine nuts is a tasty and wholesome choice for anyone on the Mediterranean diet. Have fun!

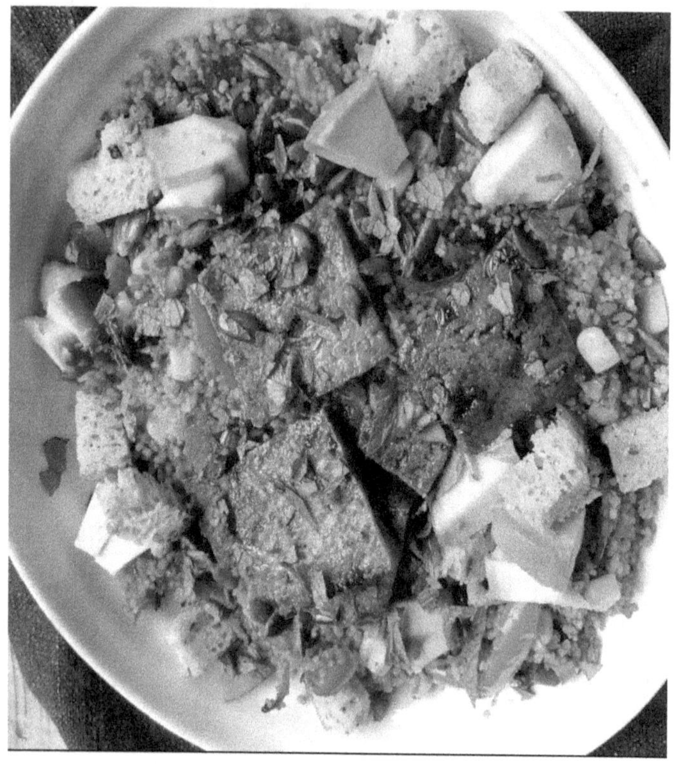

Desserts

The following dessert recipes aligns with the guidelines of the Mediterranean diet:

Fresh Fruit Sorbet

This is a straightforward recipe for Fresh Fruit Sorbet that fits into the Mediterranean diet:

Ingredients:
Two cups of a mixture of fresh berries, including raspberries, blueberries, and strawberries
1/4 cup honey and 1 tsp freshly squeezed lemon juice
half a cup of water

Instructions:
1. Clean and chop the fresh berries.

2. Place the berries, honey, and fresh lemon juice in a blender.

3. Blend until smooth, gradually adding water to get the right consistency.

4. Taste the mixture and, if necessary, add additional honey to balance the sweetness.

5. Transfer the mixture to a shallow dish and freeze it for four to six hours, breaking up the ice crystals with a fork every hour.

6. The sorbet is prepared for serving when it reaches a solid, scoopable consistency.

Savor your revitalizing Fresh Fruit Sorbet with a Mediterranean flair!

Olive Oil and Orange Cake

Here's a quick recipe for Orange Cake with Olive Oil that fits the Mediterranean diet:

Ingredients:
Two cups of all-purpose flour
One cup of extra virgin olive oil
4 big eggs and 1 cup honey
One cup of orange juice, freshly squeezed
two oranges' zests
One tsp baking powder
One-half tsp baking soda
Half a teaspoon of salt

Instructions:

1.Set the oven temperature to 350°F, or 175°C. Oil and dust a cake pan.

2. Combine the eggs, honey, and olive oil in a big basin and whisk until thoroughly mixed.

3. Include the orange zest and juice and thoroughly combine.

4.Combine the flour, baking soda, baking powder, and salt in a another basin.

5. Add the dry ingredients to the wet components gradually and stir just until incorporated.

6. Transfer the batter onto the ready pan, making sure the surface is level.

7.Place the toothpick in the center and bake for 35 to 40 minutes, or until it comes out clean.

8. After letting the cake cool in the pan for ten minutes, move it to a wire rack to finish cooling.

Savor this delectable Olive Oil and Orange Cake with a Mediterranean flair!

Honey and Nut Baklava

Here's a straightforward recipe for Mediterranean-inspired Honey and Nut Baklava:

Ingredients:
1 package phyllo dough, 1 cup melted unsalted butter, and 2 cups finely chopped mixed nuts (almonds, pistachios, and walnuts).
one tsp finely ground cinnamon
One cup of honey
half a cup of water
One tsp vanilla essence
one lemon's zest

Instructions:
1.Set the oven temperature to 350°F, or 175°C.

2. Combine the ground cinnamon and chopped nuts in a bowl. Put aside.

3. Use melting butter to brush a baking dish. Spoon additional melted butter over the phyllo dough sheet that has been laid out in the dish. Continue adding layers after that.

4. Cover the phyllo with a thick layer of the nut mixture.

5.Repeat stacking with melted butter and phyllo, adding extra nut mixture in between each time, until all of the nut mixture is utilized.

6. Add a top layer of phyllo sheets and liberally brush each layer with butter to finish.

7. Cut the baklava into square or diamond shapes using a sharp knife.

8. Bake for 30 to 40 minutes, or until crisp and golden brown, in a preheated oven.

9. In a saucepan, mix honey, water, vanilla extract, and lemon zest while the baklava bakes. Over medium heat, bring to a simmer; after that, lower the heat and simmer for ten to fifteen minutes.

10. Immediately after removing from the oven, top all of the pieces of the hot baklava with the honey mixture.

11. To allow the flavors to mingle, let the baklava cool fully before serving.

Savor this mouthwatering Honey and Nut Baklava while adhering to a Mediterranean diet!

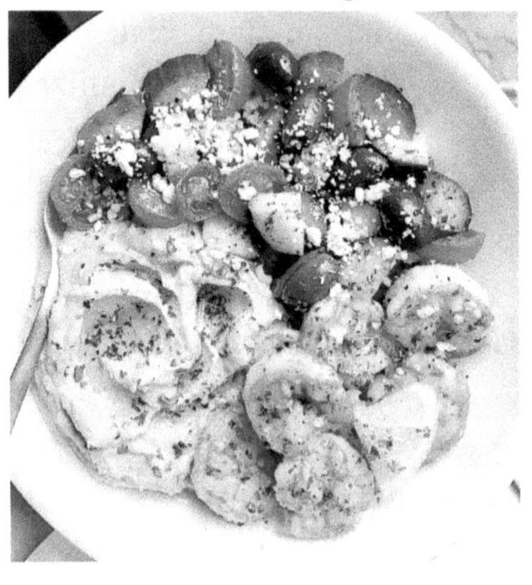

Lifestyle Tips

Keep in mind that every person has different needs, therefore customize the Mediterranean diet to your tastes and medical needs.

Tips for Grocery Shopping

The following advice can be used when grocery shopping for a Mediterranean diet:

1.Fresh Produce: Fill up on vibrant fruits and veggies, such as leafy greens, cucumbers, tomatoes, and olives. The cornerstones of a Mediterranean diet are these.

2. Whole Grains: Opt for whole grains like quinoa, brown rice, and whole wheat bread. They are nutritious and fiber-rich.

3. Lean Proteins: Choose protein sources that are low in fat, such as poultry, fish, and lentils. Salmon and other fatty fish are especially good because they contain omega-3 fatty acids.

4.Healthy Fats: Consume foods high in nuts, seeds, and olive oil, among other healthy fats.

An essential component of the Mediterranean diet is extra virgin olive oil.

5. Dairy: Include modest servings of low-fat dairy products, such as feta cheese and Greek yogurt.

6. Herbs and Spices: To enhance flavor without using too much salt, keep a supply of herbs and spices on hand, such as basil, oregano, garlic, and rosemary.

7. Canned Goods: Stock up on canned tuna, tomatoes, and beans for easy meal prep.

8. Legumes and almonds: For protein, fiber, and good fats, include a range of beans, lentils, and almonds.

9. Wine (Optional): If you're an alcoholic, think about consuming red wine in moderation. It is a staple of the diet known as the Mediterranean.

10. Cut Back on Processed Foods: Cut back on sodas, sugary snacks, and processed foods. Choose whole, less processed foods for greater health advantages.

Recall that the Mediterranean diet encompasses not just specific foods but also a whole eating habit. Place an emphasis on diversity and savor a well-balanced assortment of various food groups.

Physical Activity and the Mediterranean Lifestyle

A balanced approach to health is emphasized by the Mediterranean lifestyle, which includes a diet high in fruits, vegetables, and olive oil. An essential component of this lifestyle is regular physical activity, which improves cardiovascular health and general well-being. Exercises that support a holistic approach to health, such as walking, swimming, and cycling, fit very well with the Mediterranean way of life.

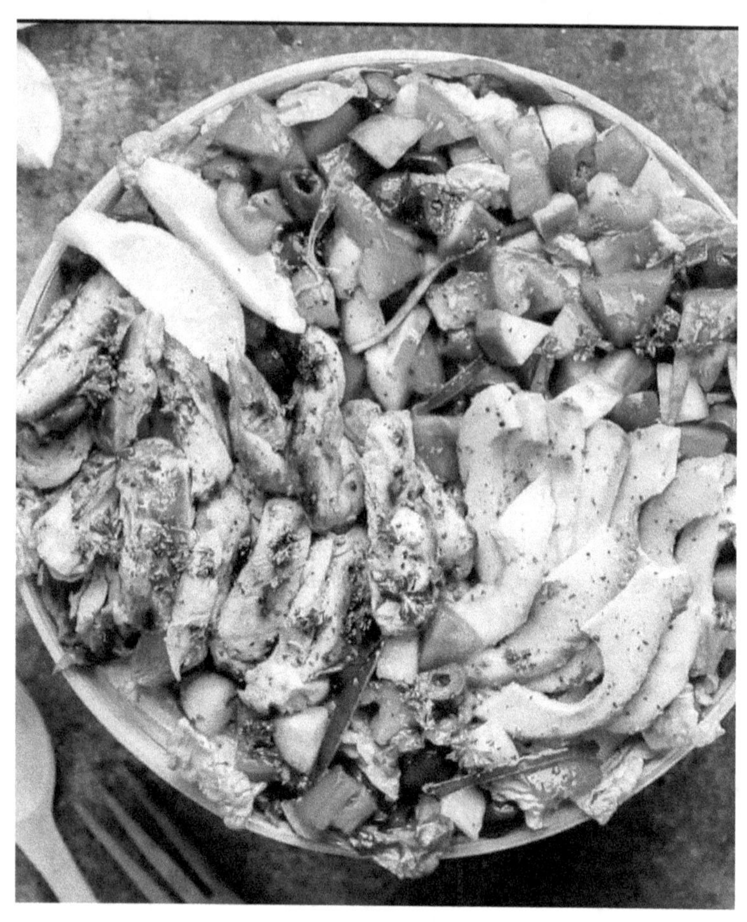

7-Days Meal Plan

This is a 7-day Mediterranean-friendly meal plan that you can adhere to:

Sample Weekly Menu

This is an example of a Mediterranean-style weekly menu:

Monday:
Breakfast:walnuts and honey with Greek yogurt
Lunch:feta cheese and a Mediterranean chickpea salad.
Dinner:grilled fish, like sea bass or salmon, topped with roasted veggies with lemon and herbs.

Tuesday:
Breakfast:avocado and tomatoes on whole grain bread.
Lunch:stuffed peppers with vegetables and quinoa.
Dinner:greek salad and chicken souvlaki with tzatziki sauce.

Wednesday:

Breakfast:oatmeal topped with almond flakes and fresh fruit.

Lunch:whole grain tortilla with hummus and veggie wrap.

Dinner:mixed greens on the side and eggplant parmesan.

Thursday:

Breakfast:smoothie that includes banana, spinach,greek yogurt, and a drizzle of olive oil

Lunch:soup with lentils and vegetables

Dinner:spaghetti with shrimp, garlic, olives, and tomatoes.

Friday:

Breakfast:feta cheese, spinach, and cherry tomatoes in a frittata.

Lunch:quinoa salad with feta, cucumber, and mint.

Dinner:rosemary-grilled lamb chops accompanied by roasted sweet potatoes.

Saturday:

Breakfast:pancakes made with whole grains and fresh fruit.

Lunch:tuna and white bean salad.

Dinner:stuffed zucchini in the Mediterranean manner with ground turkey and seasonings.

Sunday:
Breakfast:greek omelet with spinach, tomatoes, and feta for breakfast
Lunch:salad of whole wheat couscous and Mediterranean veggies.
Dinner:steamed broccoli with baked cod with lemon and capers.

Throughout the week, don't forget to include lots of fruits and vegetables, nuts, seeds, and olive oil. Adapt serving sizes to each person's specific dietary requirements.

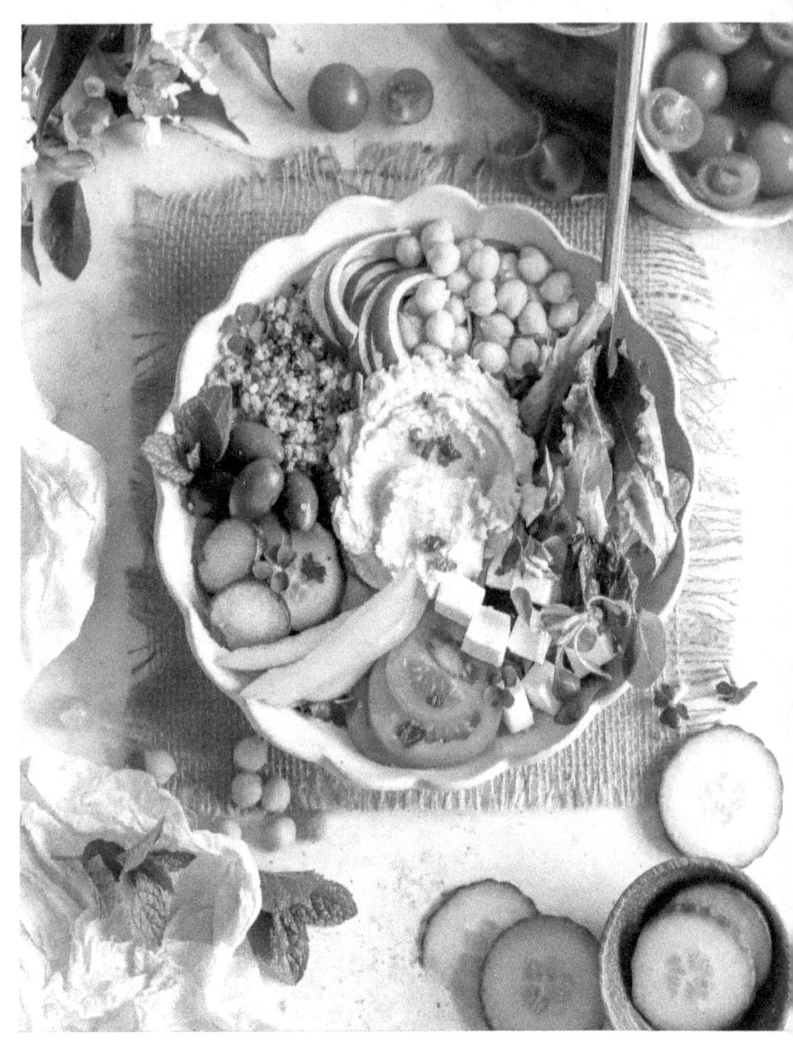

Conclusion

To sum up, the cookbook for the Mediterranean diet provides a tasty exploration of a varied and heart-healthy food world. Fresh fruits, vegetables, olive oil, and lean proteins are prioritized, and this results in tasty recipes that support a healthy, well-rounded lifestyle. This cookbook provides a guide to enjoying the many customs and well-being advantages of a Mediterranean diet, regardless of your level of culinary expertise.

Encouragement for a Healthier Lifestyle

A Mediterranean diet is a great option for leading a healthier lifestyle! Abundant in fruits, vegetables, whole grains, and good fats, this method offers a tasty and long-lasting manner to fuel your body. Recall that gradual, consistent changes result in enduring habits. Savor the bright tastes and wide variety of foods while you travel the path to improved health!

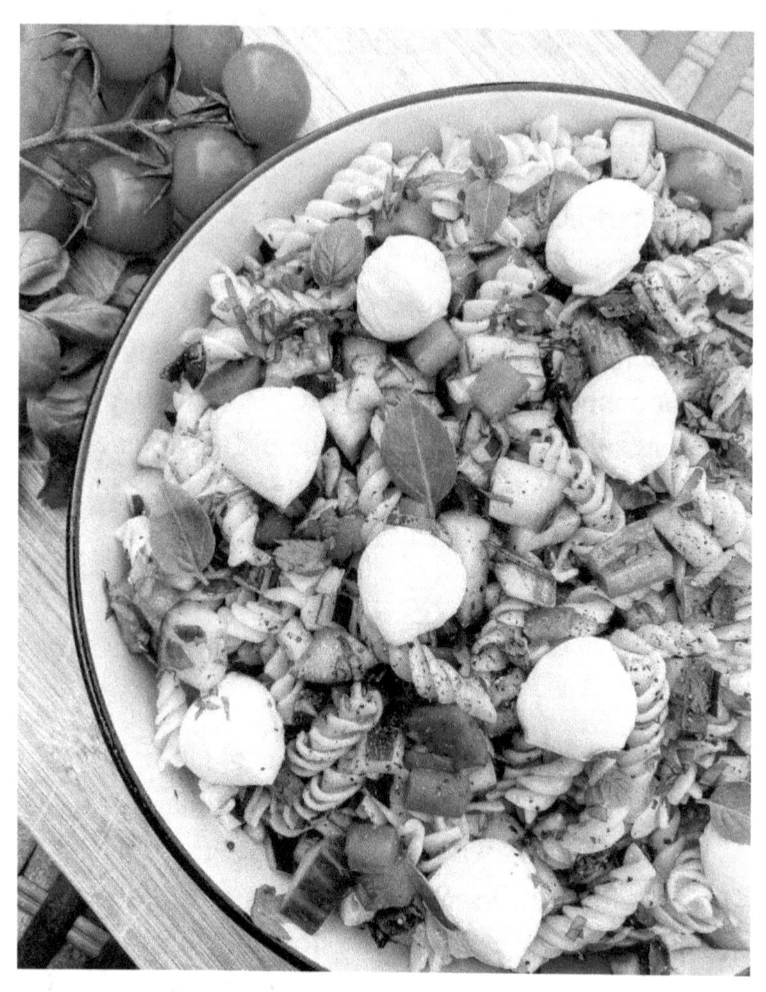